Apple Cider Vinegar
The Miraculous Natural Remedy!
Holistic Solutions & Proven Healing *Recipes*
for
Health, Beauty and Home!

by Elena Garcia

TABLE OF CONTENTS

From the Author 1

Apple Cider Vinegar- Introduction.. 2

Chapter One Health Benefits and Uses of Apple Cider Vinegar 5

Apple Cider Vinegar for Tummy Trouble and Digestive Concerns: 5

Apple Cider Vinegar to Help Ease and Cure Hiccups: 6

Apple Cider Vinegar to Sooth a Sore Throat: 7

Apple Cider Vinegar to Lower Blood Cholesterol: 7

Apple Cider Vinegar to Prevent Indigestion: 8

Apple Cider Vinegar to Clear a Stuffy Nose: 9

Apple Cider Vinegar to Aid in Weight Loss: 10

Apple Cider Vinegar to Help in the Treatment and Prevention of Dandruff: 12

Apple Cider Vinegar to Help Clear Acne: 13

Apple Cider Vinegar to Boost Energy: 14

Apple Cider Vinegar to Help with the Reduction of Nighttime Leg Cramps: 16

Apple Cider Vinegar to Help Cure Bad Breath: 17

Apple Cider Vinegar to Help Whiten Teeth: 17

Apple Cider Vinegar to Help Fade Bruises: 19

Apple Cider Vinegar to Help Control Blood Sugar Levels: 19

Apple Cider Vinegar to Help Clear up Yeast Infections: 20

Apple Cider Vinegar to Treat Foot and Skin Fungal Infections: 21

Chapter Two Side-Effects and Precautions to Consider When Using Apple Cider Vinegar 23

Chapter Three: Apple Cider Vinegar Uses in the Home............... 27

Apple Cider Vinegar to Clean and Sanitize Electronic Equipment: 28

Apple Cider Vinegar to Remove Sticky Residue from Household Scissors: 28

Apple Cider Vinegar to Remove Candle Wax: 29

Apple Cider Vinegar to Remove Ink Stains:...............................30

Apple Cider Vinegar to Clean and Unclog Household Drains:..30

Apple Cider Vinegar to Remove Mildew from the Bathroom:.... 31

Apple Cider Vinegar to Remove Mildew from your Shower Curtain: 32

Apple Cider Vinegar to Clean Out Your Washing Machine:...... 33

Apple Cider Vinegar to Freshen Up Clothes that Have Been in Storage: 33

Apple Cider Vinegar to Help Sanitize Clothes and Very Dirty Garments: 34

Apple Cider Vinegar to Help Remove wrinkles from Clothes: ..35

Apple Cider Vinegar to Clean your Iron:..................................36

Apple Cider Vinegar to Remove Stains from Porcelain Sinks and Bath Tubs:...36

Apple Cider Vinegar to Remove Greasy Residue from your Stove Top and Kitchen Counters:... 37

Apple Cider Vinegar to Remove Water Stains from Wooden Furniture:...38

Apple Cider Vinegar to Clean and Freshen Carpets: 39

Apple Cider Vinegar to Clean Stainless Steel Sinks and Cookware: 39

Apple Cider Vinegar to Polish Silver: 40

Apple Cider Vinegar to Help Prevent Spots on Your Wineglasses: 41

Apple Cider Vinegar to Remove Stubborn Coffee and Tea Stains from Coffee Mugs and Tea Cups:...41

Apple Cider Vinegar for Cleaning and Disinfecting Cutting and Chopping Boards:... 42

Apple Cider Vinegar to Clean and Deodorize your Refrigerator: 43

Chapter Four Apple Cider Vinegar for Beauty and Cosmetic Uses 45

Apple Cider Vinegar for Shiny Hair:.. 46

Apple Cider Vinegar as a Facial Mask: 47

Apple Cider Vinegar for a Detoxifying and Moisturizing Bath Soak: 48

Chapter Five Apple Cider Vinegar Recipes 49

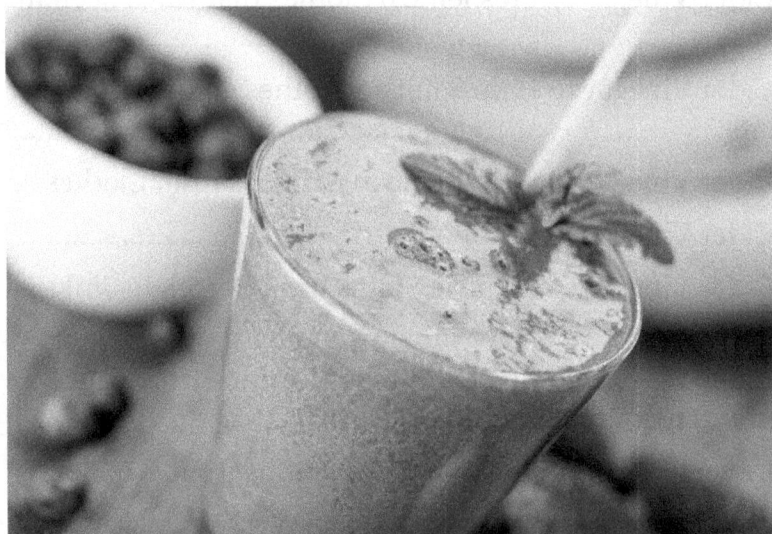

.... 49

Potassium Punch Smoothie 49

Apple Cider Vinegar Salad Dressing...51

Carrot, Orange and Apple Cider Vinegar Juice 53

Fresh Ginger Preserved in Apple Cider Vinegar.........................55

Conclusion: 57

From the Author

Thank You for taking an interest in my book. It really means a lot to me. In appreciation, I would like to offer you a free complimentary PDF eBook.

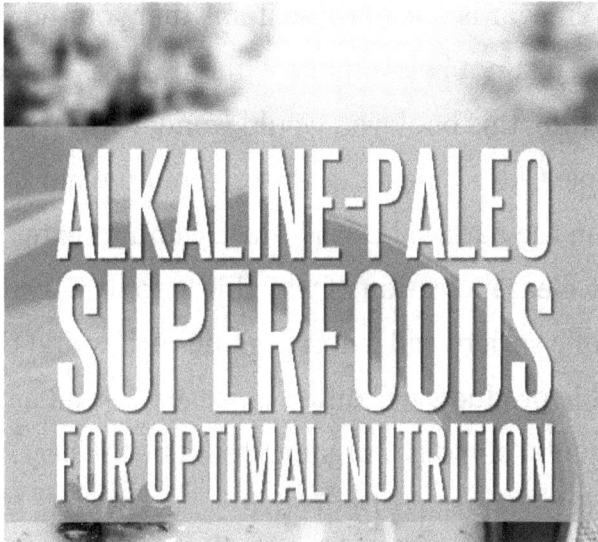

ALKALINE-PALEO
SUPERFOODS
FOR OPTIMAL NUTRITION

Tips & Recipes to Help You Thrive!

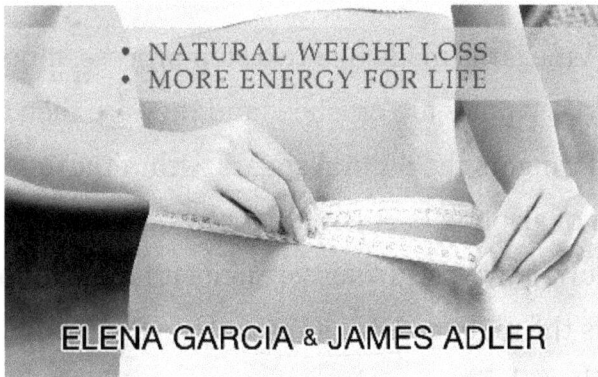

• NATURAL WEIGHT LOSS
• MORE ENERGY FOR LIFE

ELENA GARCIA & JAMES ADLER

Sign Up Link: www.YourWellnessBooks.com/email-newsletter

Apple Cider Vinegar- Introduction

Apple Cider Vinegar is one of those items that your home and kitchen would just not be complete without. It has so many uses that after reading this book you would wonder why you never tried it before. Apple Cider Vinegar is one of, if not the most popular vinegar within the natural health industry and its extensive benefits are a clear indication of why this is so. It is available in both an organic variety and a non-organic variety and the quality of the available products will differ, however they all have the same uses and benefits; obviously organic would be the best choice, but not necessarily the most cost-effective.

Apple Cider Vinegar is made in a two step process, much like most vinegar, first the apples are crushed, and they are then exposed to yeast which ferments the natural sugars within the apples causing a production of alcohol. Bacteria are then added to the now alcoholic solution, which further ferments it turning it into acetic acid, which is the main active compound in all vinegars. The organic, unfiltered varieties also contain proteins and enzymes that give the vinegar a murky appearance, thus the less clear the appearance of the vinegar, the more organic and less filtered it will be. The unfiltered varieties are also known to contain what is referred to as the "mother strand" which is what gives the vinegar a cob-web-like appearance. The mother of vinegar is composed of a form of cellulose and acetic acid bacteria which forms as a result of the fermenting of alcoholic liquids; therefore it would form during the process of adding bacteria to the crushed apple and yeast base that begins the making of Apple Cider Vinegar.

Apple Cider Vinegar is very low in calories; containing only three calories per tablespoon (15ml). Apple Cider Vinegar doesn't boast a decent content of vitamins and minerals, however it does contain a small amount of potassium, which is incredibly important for muscle recovery and many other functions within the body. Thus, as far as nutrition is concerned, Apple Cider Vinegar doesn't come to the party, however since it is known for, and celebrated, for so many other reasons it could be argued that it is still an ingredient that would be a necessity to any shopping list.

This book aims to show and enlighten you to all of the uses and benefits of Apple Cider Vinegar in terms of health and wellness, treating ailments, home use, beauty use and an extra section that includes recipe ideas that will help you further incorporate Apple Cider Vinegar into your daily routine. The side-effects and precautions of using Apple Cider Vinegar will also be explored and noted within its own chapter in order to make sure that you will be using and incorporating this vinegar into your regular routine without putting yourself at any risk or creating any harm to your health or body, so it will be important to take note of the chapter that deals with this related topic.

Chapter One
Health Benefits and Uses of Apple Cider Vinegar

Apple cider vinegar has a number of uses in terms of health, healing and remedies. This chapter will explore all of these benefits and uses and aims to enlighten you to this incredibly useful and cost effective source of natural healing. It is important to note that the chapter to follow will look at the possible side-effects and precautions of using apple cider vinegar as a treatment and remedy for health issues and preventative measures, therefore it is suggested that one reads both chapters before beginning the use of apple cider vinegar for such purposes.

Apple Cider Vinegar for Tummy Trouble and Digestive Concerns:

If you are suffering from diarrhea that is caused by a bacterial infection, the natural antibiotic and anti-bacterial properties of apple cider vinegar will make this home remedy a great option when looking to treat the symptoms of such and infection without the use of an over the counter chemical based drug. Apple cider vinegar is also known to help ease the spasms and stomach cramps that generally come with such an infection, this is a result of the high pectin content that apple cider vinegar is known to contain. To use apple cider vinegar as a remedy in this instance you would mix one tablespoon (15ml) of apple cider vinegar into one cup (250ml) of water or clear apple juice; this mixture should be sipped slowly so as not to upset the stomach an further.

Apple Cider Vinegar to Help Ease and Cure Hiccups:

Hiccups can be triggered by a number of things such as drinking alcohol, smoking, having a bloated stomach, eating too fast or eating foods that are too spicy, consuming fizzy drinks or emotions such as stress, fear or excitement. Hiccups are a result of an irritation and upset to the natural movement of the diaphragm, causing it to suck in air as it closes. This air causes the diaphragm to pull down with a jerk causing air to be sucked into the throat; the actual hiccup happens when this air rushes back up the esophagus and hits into the vocal chords. To use apple cider vinegar as remedy for hiccups take one tablespoon (15ml) of neat apple cider vinegar as you would drink cough mixture. The apple cider vinegar works in this instance because its high acetic acid content will overstimulate the throat resulting in the relaxing of the nerves within the throat that are causing the spasms that are resulting in the hiccup motion.

Apple Cider Vinegar to Sooth a Sore Throat:

A sore throat can be a result of a number of things, but the most common cause is generally a post nasal drip that can be the result of a mild sinus infection or head cold. Bacteria containing mucus drips down the back of the throat cavity causing the throat to become inflamed and painful. The anti-bacterial and antibiotic properties of apple cider vinegar make it a very useful natural home remedy for this particular health concern. To use apple cider vinegar to treat a sore throat mix ¼ cup (60ml) apple cider vinegar into ¼ cup (60ml) warm water and gargle with this solution on an hourly basis until you no longer feel that scratchy pain when swallowing. If symptoms persist and you still have a sore throat after forty eight hours of using this home remedy, it is then recommended that you consult with your doctor as you may have a more severe infection that possibly requires a harsher treatment.

Apple Cider Vinegar to Lower Blood Cholesterol:

Unfortunately there is not a lot of backing evidence and research into the theory that apple cider vinegar can indeed lower blood cholesterol. However there have been studies conducted that revealed a noted drop in the blood cholesterol levels of people who participated in the study; these participants consumed one tablespoon (15ml) of apple cider vinegar per day over the course of the study. It must be noted that blood cholesterol levels are linked to many chronic diseases and there is no single cure for it; the best way to create and maintain a healthy blood cholesterol level is by making sure that you are living a healthy, well-balance lifestyle that includes a balanced diet and sufficient exercise. It is recommended that if you have a family history of high blood cholesterol you should have your levels checked at least every one to two years and the most accurate form of testing is a fasting blood test. If you predict that you may have, or you know that you do have, high blood cholesterol levels then it is highly recommended that you consult with your physician regarding this; also it is not recommended that you pursue treatment of this concern using apple cider vinegar without consulting with your physician first.

Apple Cider Vinegar to Prevent Indigestion:

Since no two human beings are completely the same; there are certain foods and food combinations that either agree or disagree with one's digestive system. There are also those special occasions such as weddings or birthday parties where we all have the tendency to over-indulge in foods that we wouldn't normally eat on a regular basis. These could be foods that are higher in salt, fat and sugar than those that we would normally consume. Some people find the consumption of very spicy food tasty, but it can cause an irritation to their digestive systems. Everyone has their own little niggle when it comes to these things. Apple cider vinegar is a great preventative measure in such instances. To use apple cider vinegar as preemptive and preventative measure when you know or suspect that you will be over indulging in foods that may cause you to be sorry a few hours afterward mix one teaspoon (5ml) of apple cider vinegar and one teaspoon (5ml) of natural pure honey into one cup (250ml) of warm water and drink this solution half an hour before your over-indulgent meal.

Apple Cider Vinegar to Clear a Stuffy Nose:

Nasal congestion and a stuffy nose that usually comes as a side-effect of the common head cold virus is caused by a bacterial infection within the nasal and sinus cavity. Such viral infections are known to hit even the healthiest of people during the change of seasons when there are a number of viral spores floating around in the air all around us. Nasal congestion and stuffy nose can be incredibly uncomfortable and irritating; it can also lead to other concerns for example, a blocked nose will lead to one breathing through their mouth since the nasal cavity does not a have free-flowing source of air. Breathing through the mouth for an extended period of time most often leads to a dry and scratchy throat which will create further discomfort. Due to apple cider vinegar's anti-bacterial and antibiotic properties as well as its high acetic acid content, together with the potassium that is is known to contain; it will help thin the mucus that is generally the cause of the nasal congestion that one would be experiencing in a case like this. To use apple cider vinegar as a natural home remedy for nasal congestion mix one teaspoon (5ml) of apple cider vinegar into one cup (250ml) of water and drink. This can be repeated three times a day. It is important to note that if symptoms of your head cold or virus persist for longer than three days there is the possibility that you may have a more severe strain of the common virus and it would be highly recommended that you consult with your physician in this case as you may need a harsher form of treatment.

Apple Cider Vinegar to Aid in Weight Loss:

The maintenance of a healthy weight and good looking body is something that we all strive for and are consistently concerned about. There are many natural forms of healthy weight loss and maintenance, and these are always the better option rather than chemical based drugs that claim to give you the quick fix that we all wish was possible. The truth is that there is no quick fix to weight loss and maintenance and that this is only achieved through a well balanced healthy lifestyle that focuses on a balanced diet and exercise regime. However there are many natural forms of help that we can call upon in order to move the process along. Apple cider vinegar helps in this instance due to its high acetic acid content which is known to suppress appetite, boost metabolism, and reduce water retention which is a common cause of a higher number on the scale. Some scientists believe that apple cider vinegar can help the body and the digestive system in the breaking down of starch and carbohydrates, allowing them to move through your system more easily and to be absorbed in a more efficient way that does not lead to fat gain.

Apple Cider Vinegar to Help in the Treatment and Prevention of Dandruff:

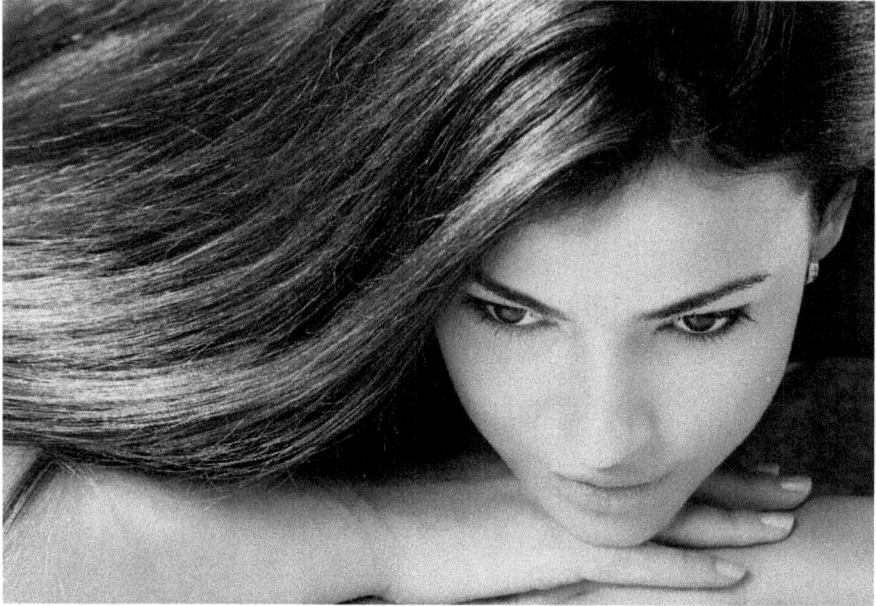

Dandruff is a common concern and many people suffer from it. The skin is the body's biggest organ and is constantly renewing and regenerating itself; as the skin renews its cells the old ones are pushed to the surface of the skin and flake off, in many people this is unnoticeable and can most likely only ever be seen on one's bath towel or face cloth. For some people this process happens at a faster rate than in others, particularly where the renewal of skin cells on the scalp are concerned. When this renewal of scalpel skin cells happens at a fast rate it results in white flakes of skin that become visible due to their accumulation in the hair, they then begin to fall to the shoulders resulting visible white flakes on your clothing; this is what is known as dandruff.

In some cases people may experience excessive flaking as a result of an underlying fungal or yeast infection. Skin conditions such as psoriasis and seborrheaic dermatitis can also lead to dandruff and excessive skin flaking.

Apple cider vinegar can help in this instance due to the fact that acidity of the vinegar changes the pH level of the skin on your scalp which will in turn make it harder for the infection-causing yeast to grow. To use apple cider vinegar as a remedy for dandruff mix ¼ cup (60ml) of apple cider vinegar with ¼ cup (60ml) of water into a spray bottle. Spray the solution generously onto your scalp before wrapping your head in a towel and allowing the solution to sit on your scalp for fifteen to twenty minutes. Wash your hair as usual and repeat this remedy twice a week.

Apple Cider Vinegar to Help Clear Acne:

In most cases severe acne is caused by an over-production of sebum by the sebaceous glands in the skin; this leads to an oilier than usual skin and can cause pimples and whiteheads, this is usually due to bacterial infection that is caused by dirt from the environment contaminating the excess sebum that is sitting on top of the skin. Very often this over-stimulation of the sebaceous glands can be induced by hormonal changes or imbalances, an irritation to the skin, or sensitivity to certain products or foods.

Apple cider vinegar can help in this instance due to its anti-bacterial and antibiotic properties which makes it a great natural and cost-effective facial toner. This is due to the malic and lactic acids that form part of the vinegar's makeup; these specific acids act as exfoliates and softeners to the skin's surface, restoring its pH balance and resulting in the reduction and treatment of red spots and their inflammation.

Apple Cider Vinegar to Boost Energy:

Intense exercise can lead to a buildup of lactic acid within the muscles of the body and this acid build up will lead to muscle stiffness and sometimes a little pain, it can also lead to both muscle and overall fatigue. This is perfectly normal and not in any way a risk, however it can become more and more uncomfortable as time goes by and that is why all professional and competing sportsmen and women all include some form of remedy for this lactic acid build-up into their daily routine.

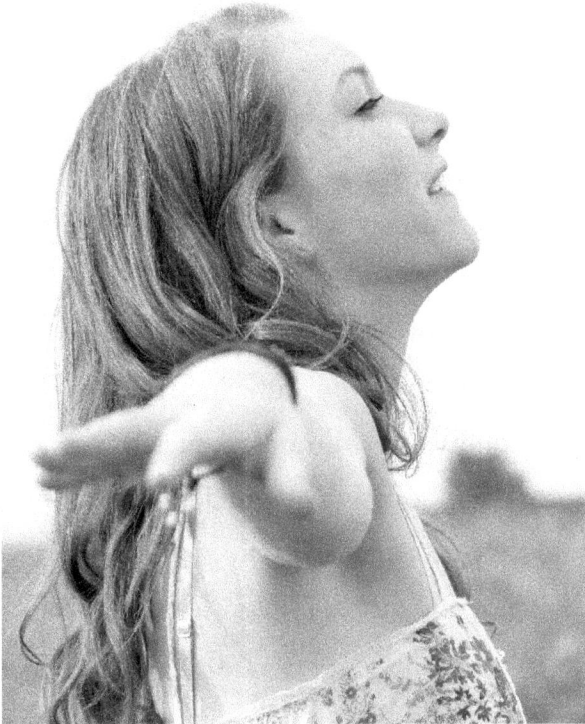

Apple cider vinegar is known to contain essential amino acids which the body uses to repair muscle fibers and boost energy levels. The potassium content in the apple cider vinegar further helps with this cause as this essential mineral is known for is potent ability to repair the normal muscle and tissue damage that comes with intense exercising; potassium is also essential in fighting both muscle and overall fatigue. To use apple cider vinegar as remedy in this instance, add one tablespoon (15ml) of apple cider vinegar to one cup (250ml) of water and drink.

Apple Cider Vinegar to Help with the Reduction of Nighttime Leg Cramps:

It's possibly safe to say that we all suffer from these excruciatingly painful leg cramps that creep up on us in the middle of the night, paralyzing your calve muscle in agonizing pain, at some point. These cramps are usually a sign that you are suffering from a deficiency in one or all of the following; sodium, magnesium or potassium. If you are sure that you body is not deficient in sodium or magnesium then the potassium content of apple cider vinegar will make it a great home remedy for this horrible, sleep disrupting cramps.

To use apple cider vinegar in this instance mix two tablespoons (30ml) of apple cider vinegar and one teaspoon (5ml) of raw organic natural honey into one cup (250ml) of warm water and drink when the cramps occur.

Apple Cider Vinegar to Help Cure Bad Breath:

Bad breath is a constant concern for all of us, and for those of us who suffer from it on a more serious level, it can be very embarrassing and can lead to one being very self-conscious. There are a number of factors that can lead to bad breath that include dental ailments, a sinus or respiratory infection, the consumption of garlic, low blood sugar levels as well as the consumption of raw onions.

Apple cider vinegar is useful as a natural remedy for bad breath due to the fact that its anti-bacterial and antibiotic properties are a great killer for bacteria that may be lurking within your mouth, causing a fowl odor. To use apple cider vinegar to treat bad breath do the following; mix one teaspoon (5ml) of apple cider vinegar with one cup (250ml) water and either gargle with this solution or drink it; how you chose to use it is completely up to personal preference.

Apple Cider Vinegar to Help Whiten Teeth:

A bright, healthy and attractive smile is something that we all want, unfortunately daily lifestyle and dietary factors can result in the yellowing or staining of teeth. These factors include smoking, the drinking of coffee and tea, as well as alcohol consumption.

Regular dental check-ups and visits to an oral hygienist on an annual basis are always recommended, but one can apply a home remedy in order to help the process undertaken by these healthcare professionals.

Apple cider vinegar is a cost-effective home remedy in this case and can be used to help whiten teeth. To use apple cider vinegar for this particular purpose gargle one tablespoon (15ml) of apple cider vinegar in the morning before brushing your teeth as usual.

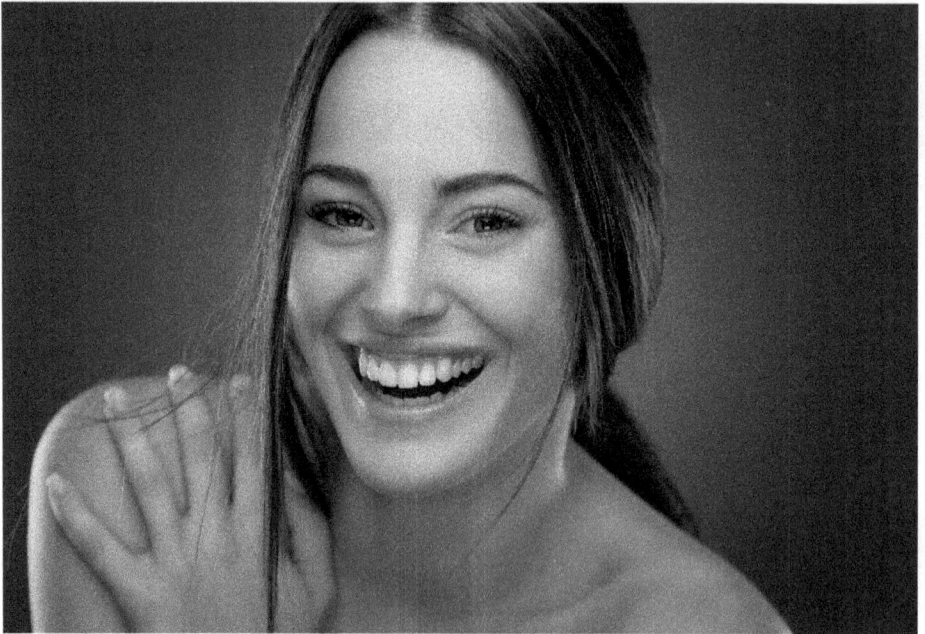

Apple Cider Vinegar to Help Fade Bruises:

Bruising is one of those unfortunate occurrences of daily life that most of us, particularly those who tend to be a little more clumsy at times, simply cannot avoid. A slight bump of the knee on your desk drawer or a bump of your elbow in passing by a doorway can lead to bruising. Bruising is usually a result of a slight bleed or burst of blood vessels underneath the skin and depending on the cause can range from minor to severe in scale. There is usually an amount of inflammation that accompanies bruising.

Apple cider vinegar can be a helpful cost-effective home remedy in this instance due to its anti-inflammatory properties. To use apple cider vinegar to help fade bruises do the following; take cotton wool padding that corresponds to the size of the bruise you want to treat, soak the cotton wool in neat apple cider vinegar and lightly compress it onto the bruise. Repeat this twice a day until the bruising has faded completely.

Apple Cider Vinegar to Help Control Blood Sugar Levels:

The maintenance of balanced blood sugar levels is important in so many ways as severe drops in blood sugar can lead to all kinds of unsavory results such as headache, nausea, fatigue; and if you are watching your weight the intense hunger that usually accompanies a severe blood sugar drop can lead to the loss of self control that results in over-indulgent eating.

If you are suffering from type two diabetes it is incredibly important to make sure that you maintain and control balanced blood sugar levels at all times. Many studies have shown a link to the home remedy of apple cider vinegar and the balancing and controlling of blood sugar levels. It is important to note that if you are aware that or you suspect that you have type two diabetes it is always highly recommended that you consult with your physician before embarking on any kind of treatment for your condition. It is also important to note that one the most effective ways of maintaining control and balance of healthy blood sugar levels is through a healthy lifestyle that includes a well-balanced diet and sufficient exercise.

To use apple cider vinegar as a means of helping to control blood sugar levels take two tablespoons (30ml) of apple cider vinegar before retiring to bed at night. One can also use apple cider vinegar as preventative measure before indulging in a high carbohydrate containing meal, that may lead to a spike in blood sugar levels; to use apple cider vinegar in this instance mix one tablespoon (15ml) of apple cider vinegar into one cup (250ml) of water and drink before your meal.

Apple Cider Vinegar to Help Clear up Yeast Infections:

A yeast infection is something that every woman will suffer from at some point in her life and is generally caused by a fluctuation in hormones, hot and sweaty environments and can also be a result of heavy sweating during exercise. Because a yeast infection is such a common medical concern it can easily be treated in a natural way.

Since apple cider vinegar has such a powerful anti-bacterial and antibiotic prevalence it is a wonderful natural remedy for treating a yeast infection. To use apple cider vinegar to treat yeast infections simply add one and a half cups (375ml) of apple cider vinegar to a warm bath and soak in the tub for approximately twenty minutes. This should be repeated once a day for the first three days of the infection.

Apple Cider Vinegar to Treat Foot and Skin Fungal Infections:

Athlete's foot is as common an infection as a yeast infection is in most people, particularly those who lead active lifestyles. Athlete's foot is commonly known as a fungal infection that affects the underside of the feet and the nail beds of the toenails; it can lead to serious discomfort and itching. Generally an anti-fungal ointment would be prescribed to treat such an infection, but these ointments are very often chemical based and can be rather harsh on the skin.

Apple cider vinegar provides a natural anti-bacterial and anti-fungal treatment for such cases. To use apple cider vinegar to treat foot and skin fungal infections you can either choose to soak the affected area in a solution of one cup (250ml) apple cider vinegar and four cups (1litre) warm water or alternatively you can apply neat apple cider vinegar directly to the affected area by soaking a cotton wool pad in the apple cider vinegar and dabbing it over the affected area.

Chapter Two
Side-Effects and Precautions to Consider When Using Apple Cider Vinegar

As with any healthcare remedy or treatment there are always significant side-effects and precautions that need to be taken into account and kept in mind at all times. Whether the treatment is natural or chemical and drug based, there are always risks involved. As mentioned in the previous chapter when using apple cider vinegar for the treatment and prevention of any medical or health problem it is always advised to seek professional medical care in the case of chronic ailments and infections.

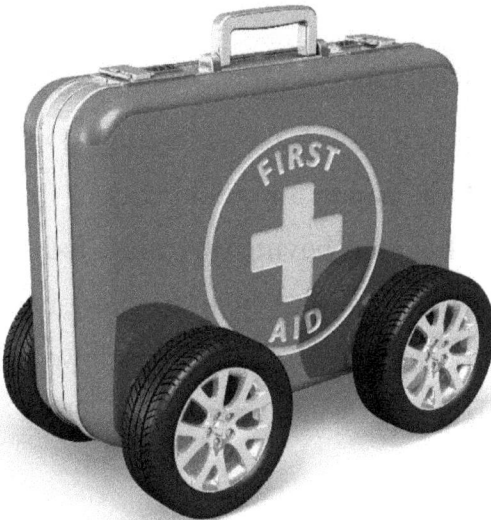

According to research and studies, the consumption of apple cider vinegar is relatively safe for most adults. However as with all natural remedies, there are some cases and instances where the use of apple cider vinegar may lead to some discomfort or complications. It has been noted that the long-term consumption of the averagely suggested one tablespoon (15ml) of apple cider vinegar on a daily basis can lead to low potassium levels within the body; this is despite the potassium content of apple cider vinegar that was mentioned in the previous chapter. According to internet research there has been one report of a case where a person developed very low potassium levels and osteoporosis, which is a chronic disease that results in very weak bones as well as the loss of bone mass; in this particular case the subject had been consuming one cup (250ml) of apple cider vinegar every day for six years.

In another report found while engaging in internet research a subject managed to get an apple cider vinegar tablet lodged in their throat, although this did not lead to any choking or asphyxiation, it was reported that after having this tablet lodged in their throat for thirty minutes, this subject began to experience pain in their voice box and reported to have trouble swallowing for up to six months after the tablet was dislodged.

It was assumed that this was a result of the high acid content of the apple cider vinegar tablet.

In terms of special precautions and warnings when using apple cider vinegar it is important to note that while pregnant and breast feeding is advised that you avoid the use of apple cider vinegar for the treatment and remedy of any ailments as there is not enough information and known side-effects or precautions regarding the use of this remedy during such a time.

When using apple cider vinegar as a means to lower and regulate blood sugar levels it is important to do so with care if you are aware of and are being treated for type two diabetes. Due to apple cider vinegar's ability to lower blood sugar levels there is a possibility that it may lower these levels to a point where they become too low and this can be incredibly dangerous if you already suffer from this chronic illness. It is also very strongly advised that you consult with your physician before beginning the use of apple cider vinegar as a remedy and treatment as it may lead to complications with your existing medical treatments and drugs.

Due to the high acid content of apple cider vinegar it is recommended that one always uses it with care and in moderation when applying it to the treatments of sore throats, teeth whitening and bad breath. There will always be the risk of over-use that can lead to discomfort and a burning of the throat and mouth due to the long-term exposure to the high acidity of the apple cider vinegar.

When using apple cider vinegar as treatment for acne, it is advised to do so with caution as well. The high acid content of the apple cider vinegar can lead to a burning of the skin if used for extended periods of time. There is also the risk of the apple cider vinegar stripping away too much of the skin's naturally occurring oils and sebum resulting in a shock effect whereby the skin will begin producing even more oil and sebum in order to protect itself from the harsh acidity of the apple cider vinegar; this could in turn cause an increase in acne and inflammation.

Once again it would be important to note that it is always a good idea to consult with a medical professional before embarking on and including the use of any home remedy or treatment whether it is in natural or chemical form.

Chapter Three:
Apple Cider Vinegar Uses in the Home

In chapter one some of the many uses of apple cider vinegar in terms of healthcare were explored. This chapter aims to show and enlighten you to the many uses of apple cider vinegar in and around the home. You will see how apple cider vinegar is incredibly useful and helpful in everyday household needs and how apple cider vinegar can be used as a cost-effective chemical free home cleaning product.

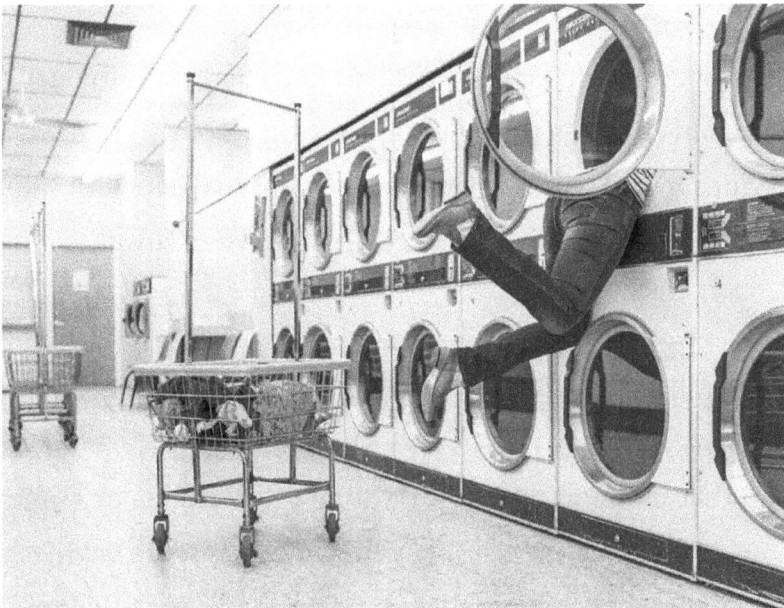

Apple Cider Vinegar to Clean and Sanitize Electronic Equipment:

This particular use applies to both home and office, so it further shows the adaptability of apple cider vinegar. Electronic equipment such as smart phones, telephones, tablets, keyboards, microwave oven buttons, printer buttons, television remote controls; any item that is used on a daily basis and is touched regularly can easily obtain a build-up of bacteria and germs over time. Since apple cider vinegar has a high acid content as well as anti-bacterial properties and due to the fact that it is a natural substance; apple cider vinegar makes a great cleanser and disinfectant for all the above mentioned electronic devices.

To use apple cider vinegar as a disinfectant and cleanser for your everyday electronic devices simply soak a cotton wool pad in neat apple cider vinegar and wipe the device you want to clean with the cotton wool pad, to dry it off use a piece of dry kitchen towel.

Apple Cider Vinegar to Remove Sticky Residue from Household Scissors:

We've all had that moment when we try to use the kitchen or home office scissors and the blades are sticky due to the scissors having been used to cut open packaging that may have had a glue sealant on it or to cut scotch tape. This can be very annoying, but apple cider vinegar is a great remedy to this because of its high acid content it is able to cut through the stickiness of the glue residue that may be on the blades of your scissors.

To use apple cider vinegar to remove glue or stickiness from your house hold scissors soak a cotton wool pad in neat apple cider vinegar and generously wipe the blades of the scissors with the cotton wool pad, making sure to remove any and all glue residue and stickiness.

Apple Cider Vinegar to Remove Candle Wax:

We all love the odd candlelit dinner and there are many occasions when the use of candles can add to the atmosphere and ambiance. There are also those times when we experience power failures and blackouts that lead to the emergency use of candles. Unfortunately due to the nature of a candle and the fact that to use it you are essentially burning and melting the wax that is it is wholly made up of; there are times when this can lead to an unwanted mess and the build-up of candle wax on the surface which you had placed the candle on. If you are using candlesticks or candle holders then there will eventually be a build-up of candle wax on these items as well.

To use apple cider vinegar to remove candle wax, heat the now hardened candle wax with a hair dryer until it has melted to a point where you can remove most of it with a cloth or a rag. There will most likely be stains and residue of candle wax left behind and this is where the apple cider vinegar comes into use. Make up a solution of one cup (250ml) of candle wax and one cup (250ml) of water, soak your cloth in this solution and rub away at the excess candle wax.

Apple Cider Vinegar to Remove Ink Stains:

One of the things that goes hand in hand with having small children around the house is that there will always be times when they disappear out of sight and get up to mischief that can lead to the unintentional defacing of household walls and floors. Almost every parent has had to, at some point, endure finding their walls to have been drawn on with pen or wax crayons and wondering just how to get rid of the stains without having repaint the house.

Apple cider vinegar is a wonderful cost-effective non-chemical way to remove such stains and to do so all you need to do is soak a cloth in neat apple cider vinegar and wipe away at the stains, you will see how they easily loosen and disappear.

Apple Cider Vinegar to Clean and Unclog Household Drains:

The clogging of household drains is something that will always eventually happen and simply cannot be completely avoided. Most of us really become concerned about a clogged-up household drain because we immediately assume that it will require a harsh chemical based product in order to help unclog and clean the drain out.

Apple cider vinegar is a great, cost-effective non-chemical way to clean out and unclog any household drain. Due to its high acid content it is able to cut through grease and detergent build-up within the drain and pipes that leads to the clogging in question. To use apple cider vinegar as means of unclogging your household drains simply mix ½ cup (125ml) of baking soda with one cup (250ml) neat apple cider vinegar and immediately pour down the clogged-up drain. The natural chemical reaction that will occur between the baking soda and the acidity of the apple cider vinegar will result in a kind of fizz-bomb that will release the drain and clean it out.

Apple Cider Vinegar to Remove Mildew from the Bathroom:

The build-up and growth of mildew in the bathroom is unfortunately another one of those household woes that we simply cannot avoid. Due to the constant dampness of a regularly used bathroom we unintentionally create a happy breeding ground for mildew, which can be very frustrating and unsightly.

Apple cider vinegar is a natural and non-chemical option for removing mildew and mildew stains from your bathroom. To remove mildew from your bathroom using apple cider vinegar mix a solution of four cups (1litre) neat apple cider vinegar to four cups (1litre) water in a spray bottle. Generously spray the apple cider vinegar solution over the mildew and allow it to sit for about twelve hours. Wash off with clean water and repeat this process as often as required.

Apple Cider Vinegar to Remove Mildew from your Shower Curtain:

The shower curtain is another happy breeding ground for mildew in the bathroom due to the way in which it tends to form folds when left open; these folds provide damp and dark crevices for the mildew to grow in and a mildew-covered shower curtain can cause many a headache on cleaning day.

To use apple cider vinegar to clean your shower curtain and remove the mildew; take the shower curtain down off the rail and place it in your washing machine. Open the detergent drawer and place ½ cup (125ml) baking soda into the wash cycle compartment and one cup (250ml) of neat apple cider vinegar into the fabric softener compartment of the detergent drawer. Run the washing machine on a full wash cycle. If possible hang the shower curtain out in full sunlight to dry once the washing machine cycle has finished.

Apple Cider Vinegar to Clean Out Your Washing Machine:

A washing machine is one of those household appliances that are used on a daily basis in most households, particularly those with large families. Over time the washing machine can fall victim to a buildup of detergent and fluff from the many loads of washing that it helps you get clean.

Apple cider vinegar is a one of the best ways to clean out your washing machine, because it is a natural substance and non-chemically based any residue of the apple cider vinegar that may remain behind in your washing machine after cleaning will not cause any potential damage or bleaching to the load of laudatory that you do afterward. To use apple cider vinegar as means of cleaning out your washing machine pour two cups (500ml) of neat apple cider vinegar into the drum of the washing machine and run it on a full cycle on the hottest temperature available.

Apple Cider Vinegar to Freshen Up Clothes that Have Been in Storage:

We all know that change of season irritation when we bring our clothes out of storage or the back of the closet only to find that they smell musty and their colors are looking a little dull. This is easily remedied by adding one cup (250ml) of apple cider vinegar to the wash cycle when washing these clothes.

Apple cider vinegar is also useful as a means of preserving and preventing the color of new clothing from running when the garments undergo their first wash. To use apple cider vinegar in this instance, soak the new garment in neat apple cider vinegar for approximately twenty minutes before washing it for the first time. This will help fix the dyes and colors within the fibers of the fabric preventing them from running and fading during future washes.

Apple Cider Vinegar to Help Sanitize Clothes and Very Dirty Garments:

Those of us who lead very active lifestyles and who regularly engage in heavy exercise sessions will know all about the effects of excessive sweating on our workout clothes. Human sweat contains odor causing bacteria and due to its high acidity content it can be rather corrosive to the fibers of that fabrics of your workout gear, and therefore needs to be successfully and completely washed out of clothes after every workout in order to preserve the life and extend the use of these particular garments.

Due to its naturally occurring anti-bacterial properties, apple cider vinegar is a wonderful cost-effective and non-chemical way of ensuring that these particular garments are well sanitized and odor free. To use apple cider vinegar in this instance simply add one cup (250ml) of apple cider vinegar to the detergent drawer when washing these clothes on a long wash cycle in the washing machine. You could also add ½ cup (125ml) of baking soda to the mix in order to ensure that all sweat stains are removed.

This mixture is also very useful as means of removing those stubborn yellow stains that tend to form around the collars and cuffs of shirts. To use the mixture for this purpose mix one cup (250ml) neat apple cider vinegar with ½ cup (125ml) baking soda into a spray bottle, generously spray the solution over the stains and allow it to sit for approximately fifteen minutes before placing the garment into the washing machine for a full wash cycle.

Apple Cider Vinegar to Help Remove wrinkles from Clothes:

If there is one household chore that is guaranteed to be everyone's worst its ironing. We all hate the idea of standing for hour upon hour at the ironing board after washing day, so any other option is always a welcome alternative.

Apple cider vinegar can help remove wrinkles from your clothes without the hardship and chore of ironing. To use apple cider vinegar as means of ironing your clothes, mix one cup (250ml) apple cider vinegar with one cup (250ml) water into a spray bottle. Spritz the wrinkled clothes with the solution and then let them hang to dry.

Chapter Three: Uses in the Home

Apple Cider Vinegar to Clean your Iron:

Unfortunately there are those fabrics that just do better once they have had good iron such as pure cotton. Over time your iron can begin to build up lime scale and dirt from general use. Apple cider vinegar is a non-chemical and cost-effective way to help clean and sanitize your iron in an easy step.

To use apple cider vinegar to clean your iron fill the iron's water reservoir with neat apple cider vinegar and then turn it onto full steam. Allow the iron to sit in the upright position steaming until all the apple cider vinegar has evaporated. Once all the apple cider vinegar has evaporated fill the iron's reservoir with clean water and repeat the steaming process.

Apple Cider Vinegar to Remove Stains from Porcelain Sinks and Bath Tubs:

Over time soap and detergent build-up can lead to stains beginning to appear on the surface and around the porcelain coating of household sinks and bath tubs. These stains can look very unsightly and cause endless frustration on cleaning day.

Harsh chemical detergents such as chlorine based household bleach can cause damage to the porcelain and over time it will cause small cracks to begin appearing in the surface of the porcelain. Although these harsh chemical products are very effective at removing stains from such sinks and bath tubs, they are also harmful to the environment and can cause skin irritations for most people.

Apple cider vinegar is a wonderful alternative to the harsh chemically abrasive detergents and is great for removing such stains. To use apple cider vinegar to remove stains from your porcelain sinks and bath tubs fill the tub or sink with hot water and add two cups (500ml) of neat apple cider vinegar. Allow to soak for approximately twenty minutes before letting the water out and wiping down with a cleaning cloth.

Apple Cider Vinegar to Remove Greasy Residue from your Stove Top and Kitchen Counters:

The buildup of a greasy residue on the stove top and kitchen counters is something that we continually try to avoid, however over time there will still be some sort of build up due to the steam and general everyday cooking within the kitchen. Chemical based detergents are not always the most desirable option to clean surfaces on which food is prepared and can in many instances cause long term damage to the coating of your stove top and kitchen counters.

Apple cider vinegar is a wonderful non-chemical and non-evasive way of cleaning and removing greasy residue from the entire kitchen. To use apple cider vinegar in this instance mix one cup (250ml) of neat apple cider vinegar with one cup (250ml) of water into a spray bottle. Spray generously over the areas of the kitchen that you would like to de-grease, allow it to sit for approximately twenty minutes before wiping off with a damp cloth.

Apple Cider Vinegar to Remove Water Stains from Wooden Furniture:

As annoying as it is and as much as we try to get our family members and regular visiting guests to use coasters there are always those moments when someone forgets to make sure there is a coaster on the table before they put their drink down. On a hot summer's day this can easily lead to the creation of a water stain that forms as a result of the condensation that builds up on the outside of a glass of cold drink; these water stains can deface your beautiful wooden furniture and cause many a heartache when trying to remove them.

Apple cider vinegar is a wonderful way to help remove such stains without resorting to re-varnishing your wood. To use apple cider vinegar to remove stains such as these from your wooden furniture soak a soft cleaning cloth in neat apple cider vinegar and rub away at the stains. Follow with a good dose of furniture polish.

Apple Cider Vinegar to Clean and Freshen Carpets:

Household carpeting regularly falls victim to the buildup of dirt and odors due to everyday accidents and general household traffic. The odd spill or muddy shoe can also lead to stains and general dirt build up on your carpeting. Due to the fact that household carpeting is made up of fibers it can also easily hold odors. The use of chemical based cleaning products in an attempt to remove these everyday stains can lead to the risk of discoloring your carpets as well as the buildup of a chemical residue that can be harmful to toddlers and crawling infants, as well as pets.

To use apple cider vinegar to clean and freshen your household carpets mix two tablespoons (30ml) of sea salt with one cup (250ml) of neat apple cider vinegar and rub over the area you would like to clean. If the area is reasonably big, double up the basic mixture accordingly. Allow the apple cider vinegar mixture to dry on the carpet and then vacuum as normal.

Apple Cider Vinegar to Clean Stainless Steel Sinks and Cookware:

Harsh water can lead to the buildup of lime scale stains on stainless steel sinks and cookware; this is due to the high lime and chlorine content that is often found within municipal water systems. These stains can be very frustrating and unsightly and very often chemical based detergents can make the problem worse.

Apple cider vinegar is a perfect non-chemical and food safe option when it comes to looking for the right product to help remove such stains. To use apple cider vinegar to remove stains from stainless steel sinks and cookware simply soak a soft cleaning cloth in neat apple cider vinegar and rub it over the stains that you are trying to remove.

Apple Cider Vinegar to Polish Silver:

We all love our silverware and those candlesticks that come out on special occasions, but it can be a serious chore to clean and polish all of these loved household items. Chemical based silverware polish tends to have a very strong odor and can lead to sinus and nasal, as well as skin irritations in most people.

Apple cider vinegar is a great non-chemical and non-irritant option for the cleaning and polishing of your silverware. To use apple cider vinegar to clean and polish your household silverware simply soak a soft cleaning cloth in neat apple cider vinegar and rub over the silverware that you want to clean and polish. If the silverware is really dirty and tarnished you can make a solution of ½ cup (125ml) apple cider vinegar and two tablespoons (30ml) baking soda, soak the silverware in this solution for about two hours and then rinse with clean water before drying off with a dry soft cleaning cloth.

Apple Cider Vinegar to Help Prevent Spots on Your Wineglasses:

There are few things more frustrating than taking out your wineglasses to set the table for a dinner party only to find that they have those annoying spots all over them that come as a result of not being dried properly after having been removed from the dishwasher. This usually results in having to spend more time "polishing" up the wineglasses with a dishcloth before setting them out on the table.

Thankfully apple cider vinegar provides an easy way to help prevent these spots from forming on the glasses in the first place. To use apple cider vinegar to prevent spots on your wineglasses simply add ¼ cup (60ml) of apple cider vinegar to the rinse cycle of your dishwasher.

Apple Cider Vinegar to Remove Stubborn Coffee and Tea Stains from Coffee Mugs and Tea Cups:

Due to the high tannin content of coffee and tea, it has a tendency to stain the porcelain on the inside of coffee and tea mugs. This is a gradual process that happens over time and long term use of the coffee and tea mugs in question. Obviously a chemical based detergent or stain remover is never going to be first choice in this instance due to the fact that they are not necessarily food safe and can cause irritations to many people's digestive systems.

Apple cider vinegar is a natural, non-chemical and very food safe option for removing these stains. To use apple cider vinegar to remove stains from your coffee mugs and tea cups simply mix one cup (250ml) of neat apple cider vinegar with one cup (250ml) of sea salt and fill each coffee mug or tea cup with a batch of this solution. Allow it to soak for about one hour before rinsing out and washing as normal. If you do have a dishwasher it would be helpful to then wash these coffee mugs and tea cups on a very hot cycle.

Apple Cider Vinegar for Cleaning and Disinfecting Cutting and Chopping Boards:

Kitchen cutting and chopping boards make for a very happy and prime breeding ground for bacteria and certain types of fungus. Making sure that your kitchen cutting boards, particularly those that are used to cut meat and fish products, are always sufficiently cleaned and disinfected is an imperative task to continually undertake in your daily kitchen habit. The buildup of bacteria and fungi within the cut grooves that form in your chopping boards with regular use can lead to a number of health problems and very often food poisoning. Any chopping or cutting board that is used to cut raw chicken needs to be thoroughly cleaned and disinfected after every use as there is always the risk of contracting salmonella from raw chicken.

Very often people will soak their chopping and cutting boards in household bleach in order to ensure that they are sufficiently cleaned and decontaminated, however this is a very harsh chemical based detergent that is not necessarily food safe and if the chopping and cutting board is not sufficiently rinsed of all excess household bleach it can also lead to the cause of discomfort and digestive upsets.

Apple cider vinegar is a natural and food safe way of disinfecting and sufficiently cleaning your kitchen chopping and cutting boards. Because of its naturally occurring anti-bacterial and antibiotic properties, apple cider vinegar provides a food safe way of cleaning these everyday kitchen items. To use apple cider vinegar to clean your chopping and cutting boards simply soak them in neat apple cider vinegar for approximately one hour and then run them through the dishwasher on a very hot cycle, alternatively soak them in boiling water for a further hour.

Apple Cider Vinegar to Clean and Deodorize your Refrigerator:

The refrigerator is another of those essential household appliances that can easily fall victim to the buildup of dirt and odors, purely due to its primary use. As much as we all try to avoid forgetting about that tub of leftovers that ends up getting pushed to the back of the fridge and going bad, it's something that happens anyway and can lead to nasty odors staying behind within the refrigerator.

Obviously since the refrigerator is where we store our food, none of us are particularly keen to jump at the chance to clean it out with a harsh chemical-based detergent. Apple cider vinegar, with its naturally occurring anti-bacterial and cleansing properties is a great non-chemical alternative to use to clean and deodorize your refrigerator. To use apple cider vinegar to clean your refrigerator simply mix a solution of equal parts of neat apple cider vinegar to plain warm water; using a cleaning cloth that you have dampened in the apple cider vinegar solution, wipe down the interior shelves and door of your refrigerator before repeating the process on the outside of the refrigerator.

Chapter Four
Apple Cider Vinegar for Beauty and Cosmetic Uses

Apple cider vinegar has many uses when it comes to beauty and cosmetic concerns and since it such a natural and safe to use product it makes a wonderful alternative to the chemical-based and highly fragranced options that the commercial cosmetic industry has to offer to us. It is however important to note that due to apple cider vinegar's high acidity content it can cause irritation and a burning sensations to very sensitive skin. This chapter aims to show and enlighten you to some of the many uses of apple cider vinegar for beauty and cosmetic related concerns.

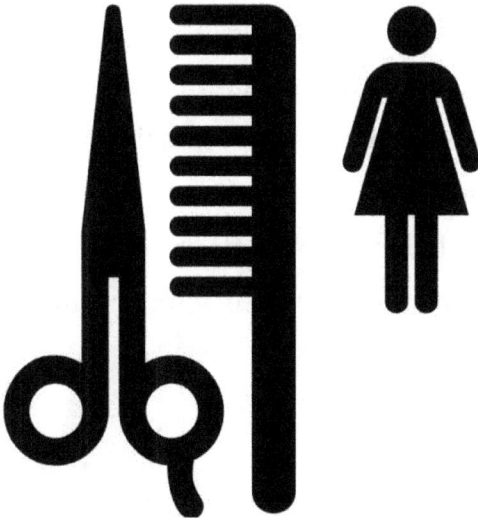

Apple Cider Vinegar for Shiny Hair:

A beautiful shiny and soft main of hair is something that we all long for and always strive to achieve within our beauty regime. Many of the products made available to us by the cosmetic industry are chemical-based and highly fragranced, which can lead to irritations for people with sensitive skin. Also the extended use of styling products can lead to a buildup of these products in our hair causing it to be weighed down and look dull and lifeless.

Apple cider vinegar has a high acetic acid content and is a natural alternative to the products made available by the cosmetic industry for such concern. The use of apple cider vinegar on your hair will naturally remove the buildup of styling products and at the same time strengthen the hair shaft, resulting in a healthy hair follicle that will in turn produce and grow a healthier, shinier strand of hair. Apple cider vinegar will also help to restore the natural pH balance of the scalp and hair shafts resulting in an increase in hair growth and volume. To use apple cider vinegar as a hair tonic dilute ¼ cup (60ml) neat apple cider vinegar into four cups (1litre) of warm water and pour this solution over your hair after shampooing. Leave the solution to sit in your hair for approximately five minutes before rinsing off with cold water, the cold water will seal the hair shaft resulting in shinier hair.

Apple Cider Vinegar as a Facial Mask:

Due to its high acetic acid content as well as its anti-bacterial properties, apple cider vinegar makes a great base for a detoxifying facial mask. The honey that is added to this mixture adds further naturally occurring anti-bacterial properties as well as moisturizing properties for the skin. This natural facial mask mixture also contains bentonite clay which is made up of volcanic ash and is celebrated for its natural detoxifying properties.

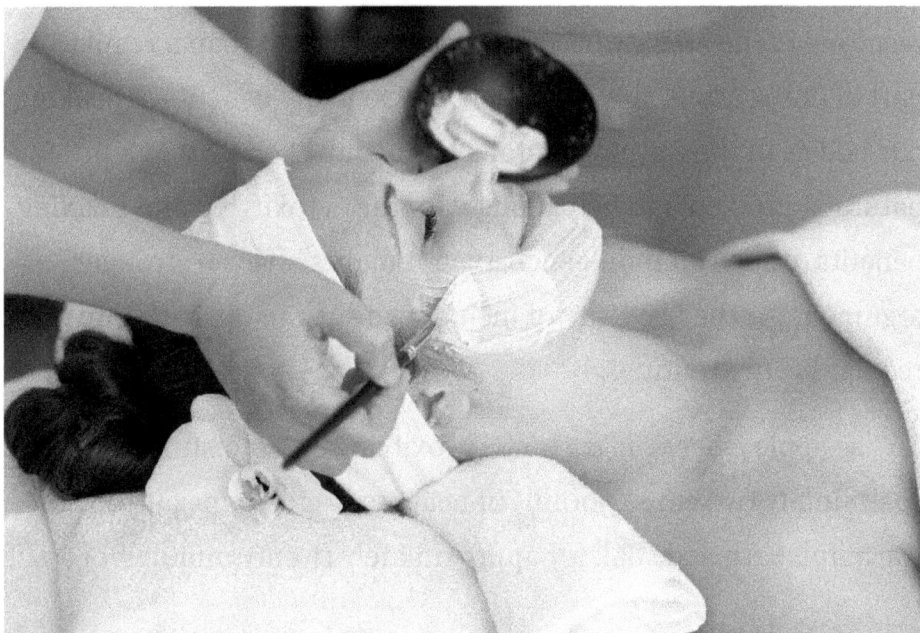

To use apple cider vinegar to make a facial mask mix one cup (250ml) neat apple cider vinegar with one cup (125ml) bentonite clay and one tablespoon (15ml) raw natural honey, make sure you combine all the ingredients into a paste. Apply the mask to cleansed skin and allow it to sit for ten to fifteen minutes before washing off with clean warm water. Pat your face dry and then soak a cotton wool pad in neat apple cider vinegar and wipe the pad over your skin, using the apple cider vinegar as a toner. Follow with your usual moisturizing routine.

Apple Cider Vinegar for a Detoxifying and Moisturizing Bath Soak:

In our fast paced modern lifestyles finding the time to indulge in the activity of soaking in a bath can be very difficult for some of us resulting in the activity becoming more of a treat than a regular part of our routine. However there are so many benefits to soaking our bodies in the warm water of a bath, and when we add a little natural ingredients to help along with the detoxifying and relaxing benefits of such an indulgence, then it makes an even stronger argument for the necessity of including a soak in the bath into our regular beauty routine.

To use apple cider vinegar for a detoxifying and moisturizing bath soak simply two cups (500ml) of neat apple cider vinegar to your warm full bath and soak for approximately twenty minutes.

Chapter Five
Apple Cider Vinegar Recipes

At the end of the day apple cider vinegar is still a food product and therefore this chapter on recipes that use apple cider vinegar even further illustrates how versatile this natural product just is. The recipes in this section will give you a few basic ideas of how to incorporate apple cider vinegar into your daily cooking routines in order to further reap the health benefits and properties that it possesses.

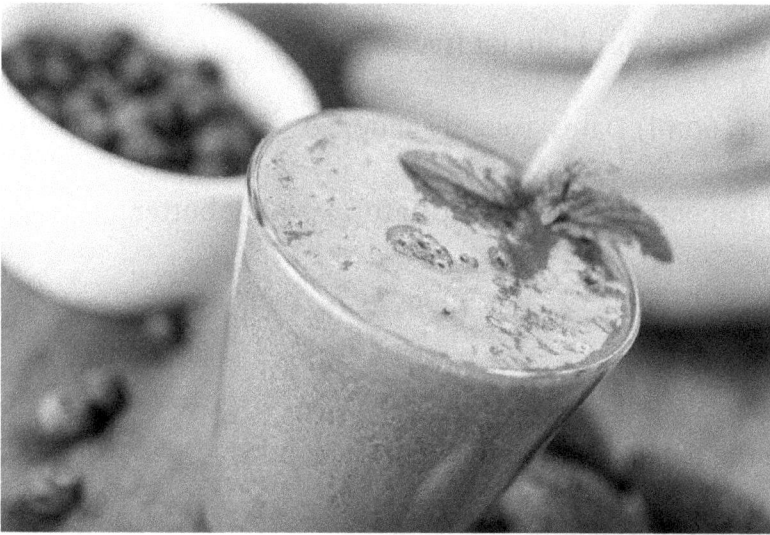

Potassium Punch Smoothie

Bananas are known for their high potassium content and are a very healthy source of easily digestible carbohydrates, making them one the best fruit options for active people and are an amazing pre and post workout food. The dates in this recipe add an extra punch of fiber and vitamin C as well as the essential mineral of iron. The potassium content of the apple cider vinegar adds the extra dose of this muscle restoring and cramp preventing essential mineral. The calcium that is brought to the party by the yogurt makes this smoothie a great source of bone strengthening ingredients as well

Serve One

Ingredients:

- One large banana

- One cup (250ml) Plain fat free yogurt

- ¼ cup (60ml) Dates, roughly chopped

- 1 Tablespoon (15ml) Organic natural peanut butter

- 1 teaspoon (5ml) Organic apple cider vinegar

Instructions:

1. Slice the banana into to the jug of a blender

2. Add the fat free yogurt

3. Add the dates and peanut butter

4. Add the apple cider vinegar

5. Blend until smooth

Apple Cider Vinegar Salad Dressing

Salad dressings don't have to be high in calories and added preservatives; they also don't have to be high in synthetic flavors and chemical additives like mono-sodium-agglutinate (MSG). This recipe will show you how to make a healthy, health benefiting salad dressing using simple and natural ingredients.

Ingredients:

- 1 Cup (250ml) Apple cider vinegar

- ½ Cup (125ml) Extra Virgin Olive Oil

- 1 Teaspoon (5ml) Organic sea salt

- 1 Teaspoon (5ml) Ground Black pepper

- 1 Tablespoon (15ml) Fresh Basil, finely chopped

- 1 Tablespoon (15ml) Fresh or dried Rosemary

- 1 Teaspoon (5ml) Red chili, seeded and finely chopped

- 1 Teaspoon (5ml) Fresh garlic, finely chopped

Instructions:

1. Place all the ingredients into a salad dressing shaker and shake vigorously making sure that you combine all the ingredients together sufficiently.

2. Pour the salad dressing into a glass jar and refrigerate

3. To use: Pour one tablespoon (15ml) of the salad dressing over your favorite salad before serving.

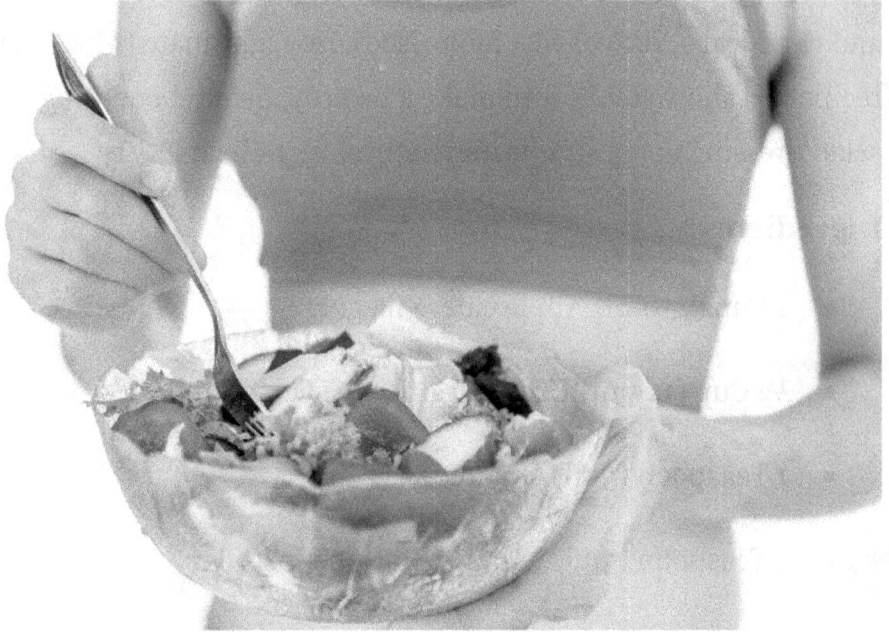

Carrot, Orange and Apple Cider Vinegar Juice

Home made fresh juices are a wonderful way to ensure that you are getting all the health benefits of the fruits and vegetables that you are consuming without any of the added preservatives that are a guaranteed part of commercially packaged juices. Over the last few years we have seen an increase in the popularity of homemade juices and this is a wonderful thing to see as it means that more and more people are taking control of their health and wellness and making sure that they always know what they are consuming. This juice combination is high in antioxidants and vitamin C from the orange juice and the carrot brings along a healthy dose of beta-carotene and vitamin A. The potassium content in the apple cider vinegar, along with its anti-bacterial and antibiotic properties as well as the addition of pure honey make this juice a wonderful idea when fighting off any infection.

Serves One

Ingredients:

- One large orange, peeled and segmented

- One large carrot

- One tablespoon (15ml) Organic apple cider vinegar

- One tablespoon (15ml) Raw organic natural honey

Instructions:

- Using a juicing machine feed the orange segments into the chute

- Feed the carrot into the chute

- Add the apple cider vinegar

- Add the honey

- Juice all together to ensure that all is mixed well

- Pour into a glass and serve.

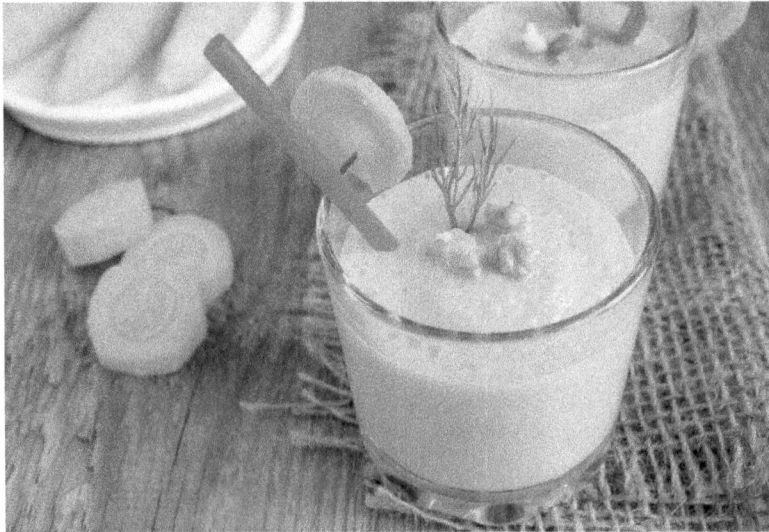

Fresh Ginger Preserved in Apple Cider Vinegar

Fresh ginger has a number of health benefits including anti-bacterial and anti-inflammatory properties. It is also an incredibly useful ingredient in so many dishes from curries to smoothies and desserts. It is always helpful to have some finely chopped ginger close on hand when you are busy preparing your favorite dishes for which ginger is a key ingredient to the overall flavor. In order to preserve the shelf and refrigeration life of pre-chopped ginger we need to add a natural form of preservative. Apple cider vinegar has a high acetic acid content, making it a great natural alternative to any commercial preservative. By adding apple cider vinegar to the jar in which you are keeping your chopped ginger you are naturally extending its shelf life.

Ingredients:

- One cup (250ml) Fresh ginger root, peeled and chunked

- One cup (250ml) Organic apple cider vinegar

Instructions:

1. Place the peeled, chunked fresh ginger root into a food processor fitted with the chopping blade

2. Pulse until the ginger is very finely chopped

3. Place the ginger into a glass jar

4. Pour the organic apple cider vinegar into the glass jar with the ginger, ensuring that all the ginger is covered with the vinegar

5. Keep in the refrigerator and use as needed.

Conclusion:

This book shows the many uses and benefits of apple cider vinegar; however since there really are so many it could be argued that this book only touches on these mentioned ways of using and benefiting from this natural product. It is once again necessary to add, in conclusion, that one must always take care when using any product as a natural remedy for health concerns and that it is always a good idea to consult with your healthcare professional before embarking on the use of apple cider vinegar for any health related issue.

PS. One more thing, before you go; could you please **rate this book on Amazon** and let me now your favorite ACV salt tip? It would be really much appreciated and would help me serve you better.

Thanks in advance,

Elena,

www.ingramcontent.com/pod-product-compliance
Lightning Source LLC
Chambersburg PA
CBHW070758300326
41914CB00053B/730